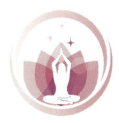

Keerthy Sunder, MD is an accomplished physician with training in Obstetrics, Psychiatry and Addiction Medicine. He earned Diplomates from the American Board of Psychiatry and Neurology in Buffalo Grove, Ill., the American Board of Addiction Medicine in Chevy Chase, Md., and the Royal College of Obstetricians and Gynecologists in London, England. He has also been certified as a Credentialed Menopause Practitioner by the North American Menopause Society, and is currently licensed by the medical boards of California, Arizona, Pennsylvania, New York and England.

Dr. Sunder served his Ob/Gyn residency at James Cook University Hospital in England. He served his Psychiatry residency at the University of Bristol, England as well as Western Psychiatric Institute and Clinic at the University of Pittsburgh Medical Center in Pennsylvania. Also, he has obtained extensive training in the practice of mind body medicine and integrative approaches towards health and wellness.

He is the Principal Investigator for Central Nervous System Clinical Trials and Medical Director for MBTRINS (Mind & Body Treatment & Research Institute) in California.

You can reach Dr. Keerthy at DrKeerthy@MBTRINS.com.
www.MBTRINS.com

Face Your Addiction
&
Save Your Life

BY: KEERTHY SUNDER, MD
MEDICAL DIRECTOR
Mind & Body Treatment and Research Institute

Copyright

Mind & Body Treatment and Research Institute
3060 El Cerrito Place Suite 266 El Cerrito, CA 94530
www.ASoundMindAndBody.com

Disclaimer

Dedication

My deepest gratitude to wonderful human beings all over the world who share their struggles and joys as they finds ways to beat their addictions one day at a time. This book is dedicated to all of you!

 I could not have accomplished this work without the incredible support from Dr. Mike Woo-Ming, Chris & Todd Huish, Rori and all the incredible support staff at Green Pixel Development and to each one of them I express my heartfelt thanks.

Table of Contents

What is Addiction?

If you asked 100 people this question, you might hear things like "a weakness," "a character flaw," "a lack of will power," "a chemical dependency," and a lot of other most likely negative answers. But you are unlikely to hear the right answer because most people don't understand that addiction, in all its forms, is a brain disease. Recent advances in the capabilities of neuroimaging have provided a new view of what causes the compulsive behaviors associated with addiction and a much clearer understanding of what is happening inside the brain that makes it so difficult to overcome.

Basically, the reason that addicts, like those that abuse opiates and other drugs, continue to participate in the compulsive behaviors associated with the disease despite the significant negative consequences that are present every time they do so, is because their brains are hard wired to keep doing them.

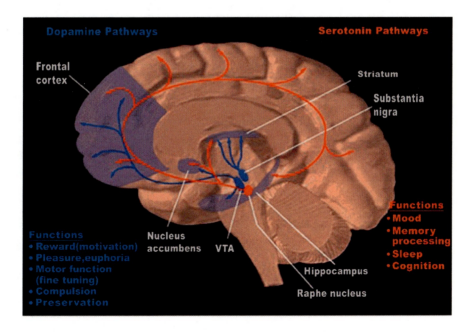

Taking drugs activates the reward system in the brain. In normal brains, this system is activated by activities like eating and having sex. When we engage in these activities the brain releases dopamine, a neurotransmitter.

The dopamine travels down previously established pathways that run between the limbic system and the hippocampus, creating a connection between our emotions and our memory. This connection is how the reward pathways for these activities, which are crucial for survival of the species, become hardwired in the brain.

When we participate in these activities, that hardwired pathway is activated, dopamine is released, and we experience pleasure. The connection between the limbic system and the hippocampus creates an association between that pleasurable reward and the memory of the activity.

This is then used by our brain to encourage us to participate in that activity again. Each time the pathways are activated, the activation reinforces that pathway, essentially hardwiring it in the brain. This reward system is evolution's way of encouraging us to engage in these activities again and again in order to ensure the continuity of the species.

Now consider what happens when drug use takes the place of sex or eating in this explanation. In essence, the drug use highjacks the hardwired dopamine pathways and makes them its own. Each time the person takes drugs, that hardwiring is reinforced and the person is encouraged, by the chemicals in their brain, to engage in using drugs again. The more the pathways are activated this way, the more hardwired they become for drug use and the harder it becomes to stop doing it, at a biological level.

This means that in order to stop using drugs, these pathways need to be reclaimed and rewired to function the way they do in a normal brain.

But there is even more to the story.

In addition to hijacking the pleasure pathways, drug use appears to have another effect on the brain that makes addiction even more challenging to overcome.

While the drugs are joyriding the brain's pleasure pathways, they are also messing around with the brakes, causing changes in how the part of the brain that keeps us from doing things with negative consequences, like drugs, functions. As the drug use increases, the part of the frontal lobes of the brain that is best equipped to stop us using inhibition and willpower, become less functional.

Scientific advances have also helped researchers understand how addicts develop what is commonly referred to as "tolerance" which requires them to take a higher dose or larger amounts of their drug of choice to get the same response. Neuroimaging shows that when the brain is frequently overloaded with dopamine, as it is for drug addicts, it will try to compensate by creating fewer dopamine receptors.

This means that even though the drug is triggering the release of dopamine, not as much of it makes it to those hijacked pathways and the reward experience is not as gratifying. However, the mechanism that encourages the drug use, that causes the craving and the compulsive need to do drugs is still activated which means addicts do more drugs in order to meet that need.

With this increased understanding of what is happening in the brain when drugs are taken, researchers and clinicians are better able to create treatment protocols and individual recovery plans that treat addiction as the disease it is.

The Basics of Addiction

As scientific studies have provided new data beneficial in building a more comprehensive understanding of addiction, doctors and researchers have been able to use that data to identify the factors that contribute to addiction. Three of these factors are a person's individual biology and genetic pre-disposition, their environment, and the effect of the drug on the brain's mechanisms.

Biology/Genetic Disposition

The individual biology of any given person, which includes their genetic make-up, plays a part in how vulnerable they are to drug addiction. Research suggests that one of the parts biology may play in addiction vulnerability relates to the number of dopamine receptors in the brain.

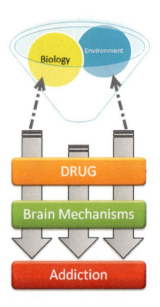

Based on the understanding of how the brain's dopamine-fueled reward system relates to all forms of addiction, researchers hypothesized that those with lower numbers of dopamine receptors may be more susceptible to the effects of drug use and therefore more vulnerable to drug addiction.

One study sought to test this hypothesis by observing how Ritalin, a medication that affects dopamine levels in the brain, affected test subjects. Each participant was given the drug and then researchers imaged their brains with a PET scan to determine their level of dopamine receptors. Participants were then asked how they felt about the effects of the Ritalin.

They found that people who had higher levels of dopamine receptors generally disliked the effects of the Ritalin while those who had low levels of receptors liked the way it made them feel. These findings suggest that differences in dopamine receptors can play a role in how susceptible an individual is to drug abuse.

Environment

Researchers have also identified that the environment in which a person grows up or lives can impact how their genes are expressed in their brain. For example, being exposed to peers who use drugs may be a risk factor for drug abuse from a psycho-social perspective, but it may also impact how the person's genes are expressed making them more vulnerable to addiction. This only underlines the complex nature of drug addiction and confirms that it is a chronic disease that must be treated as we would treat Hypertension or Diabetes.

Addiction is Like Other Diseases

For years, drug addiction has been seen as a problem caused by drugs. Under this paradigm, people became addicted to drugs because they chose to use drugs and to continue using drugs. That choice was seen by society as a selfish, reckless choice made by people who were then vilified for their lack of morality and weak willpower. This paradigm also considered access to drugs to be a significant part of the problem. From this standpoint, if access were eliminated, the problem would disappear. The vilification of addicts and societal pressure to eliminate access gave us the War on Drugs, the U.S.'s $1 trillion dollar failed campaign to end drug use and abuse.

But addiction is not the result of weak morals, lack of willpower, or easy access to drugs. It is a disease and just like other diseases, people don't choose to get it. It is preventable. It is treatable. But in order to treat it, we have to understand it. We have to understand the biological changes resulting from drug abuse and how to counteract or treat them. We need to understand what makes this person become an addict rather than that person. And most importantly, we need to change how everyone, from addicts to law enforcement to family members to society as whole, sees drug addiction and those who suffer from it.

Addiction Changes Your Biology

For years, the medical establishment has known that drug abuse can cause permanent damage to the brain. But until recent advances in neuroimaging, the full effects of drug abuse on the brain were not even theorized. These advances are completely changing the understanding of addiction and the biological changes and factors in play.

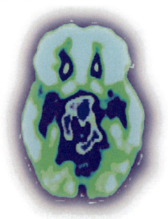
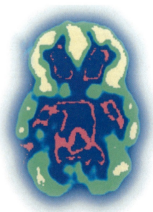

HEALTHY BRAIN   ADDICTED BRAIN

"Positron emission tomography (PET) and Fluoro-2-deoxyglucose (FDG–PET) measure glucose metabolism, which is a sensitive indicator of damage to the tissue in the brain. Decreased glucose metabolism in the OFC (orbitofrontal cortex) of the addicted brain results in improper inhibitory control and compulsive behavior. Abnormalities in the OFC are some of the most consistent findings in imaging studies of addicted individuals (including alcoholics) although they are not detected in all addicted individuals."

One of the most important things research has shown in recent years is how drug abuse affects the brain. As explained above, using drugs affects how the brain works, hijacking pleasure pathways and rendering inhibitory control and willpower ineffective. And this research is only the beginning. Even though there is still much we don't know, the fundamental shift in understanding that is moving addiction from a lifestyle choice to a disease has opened the door to new ways of thinking about how biology and addiction are interconnected that can only make prevention and treatment more effective in the future.

Addiction is Preventable

After decades of anti-drug programs aimed at preventing people from using drugs, the rate of illicit drug use and the number of people addicted to drugs remains high. Years of anti-drug taskforces and mandatory minimum sentences for drug related crimes have filled our prisons but seem to have had little effect on the rate of drug use or the number of addicts. Families have struggled for years and spent tens of thousands of dollars on treatment plans attempting to help drug-addicted family members overcome their addiction, only to lose those family members to what was considered a self-inflicted wound.

All of this has led to the widespread belief that drug addiction is not something that can be prevented. But the truth is that drug abuse can be prevented, if we are using the right kind of preventative methods. The efforts of the past failed not because it is an impossible task but because the methods used for prevention and treatment were based on a flawed understanding of what was causing the addiction in the first place.

Addiction is Treatable

Thankfully, there have been persons afflicted with addiction who were able to overcome their addiction with the use of 12 step programs or other support structures and went on to live productive drug-free lives. Unfortunately, this is more often the exception than the rule. Many more people are never able to overcome their addiction and most of those that do relapse, often repeat the cycle of rehab to relapse again and again. This has created a misconception that treatment for drug abuse works based on the willingness, moral fortitude, and strength of character of the addict. In other words, if treatment doesn't cure your addiction or you relapse, it was because you weren't trying hard enough or you weren't committed enough. It was your fault if you relapsed.

But this misconception is also based on the flawed premise that addiction is not a disease, but a lifestyle choice. No one has ever looked at a cancer survivor who has come out of remission and told them the cancer only came back because they didn't try hard enough to live cancer free. But this is exactly what happens to drug addicts.

Additionally, when research indicated that drug abuse caused brain damage, the belief that this brain damage was irreversible and made treatment impossible was born. But the truth is that the way we have been treating drug addiction simply isn't adequate, effective, or sufficient. These methods were often unhelpful, useless, and in some cases, harmful to those that they were trying to help.

Changing the way we treat drug addiction is the key to recovery and restoration of health. Research into addiction as a disease has opened the door to the development of new treatment methodologies that offer hope for addicts and their families. As our understanding of the biology behind this disease improves, so will our ability to create new and even more effective ways of treating the disease and helping those who have it live healthy lives again.

How Addiction Happens

Triggers, Cravings, Relapse

Earlier you read about how the brain becomes hardwired and compels the addict to continue using drugs. Once that hardwiring is in place, the mechanism the brain uses to create that compulsion is called a trigger.

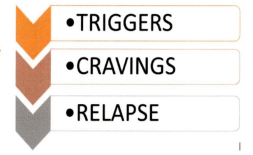

These are the thoughts, feelings, experiences, and sense memories that make the addict want to take drugs. In essence, when a trigger is activated it causes a craving. This craving is the driving force behind the compulsive need to use drugs.

There are different kinds of triggers. Internal triggers are generally related to emotions, most commonly unpleasant, uncomfortable, or negative emotions like shame, fear, guilt, anxiety, depression, and anger. External triggers are generally related to things like places, people, events, and sensory inputs.

In a perfect world, the cure for addiction might be removing these triggers or permanently shielding the addict from them, but neither of those things is possible. This means that curing addiction has to take into account that being exposed to these hardwired triggers is unavoidable.

One of the ways that addicts can control their drug use is to identify these triggers, learn to catch them as they are occurring, and then find ways of stopping the trigger from activating so that the craving is never created. But the trigger remains in place which means the addict always runs the risk of missing the activation of a trigger or failing to stop one before it causes a craving which almost inevitably leads to a relapse of drug use.

Research indicates that the most crucial time for addicts in recovery comes between 30 and 90 days of being clean. This is when triggers are the most prevalent and active and other issues that make sobriety so difficult are at their peak.

Once that 90 day milestone is reached, the ability to disable triggers, resist cravings, and remain drug-free increases day by day. But in order for that to happen, addicts must learn the techniques, strategies, and tricks, know their triggers and stop them from causing cravings very early in the process.

What's True and What's Not

The shifting paradigm about the nature of drug addiction means many misconceptions remain about what causes people to become addicted. Part of changing this paradigm is correcting these misconceptions.

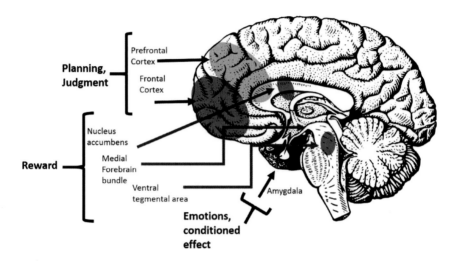

For addicts and those who love them, the most important truth that must be embraced is that addiction is a disease.   It is not a choice. It is not a character flaw. And it cannot be "cured" by being strong or by sheer force of will. It can, however, be prevented and it can be treated. Addiction can't be treated with tough love and it is not a bad habit that can be "kicked" simply because the person wants to be drug-free bad enough. It is a disease. It needs to be treated with medication, with evidence-based counseling, and with love and support from family and friends.

Treating addiction with medication is about recovering from addiction. Unfortunately, many addicts and their family, friends, and even society believe this means replacing an addiction to one drug with an addiction to a new drug. But this is simply not true. Medication used to treat drug addiction is used to create a safe environment where the addict can do the work required to overcome their addiction.

Addicts need this support so that they can learn what they need to know to identify their triggers and stop their cravings. Without it, they have to battle the very things they are trying to learn to control. It would be like trying to teach someone to walk again after an injury without giving them any railings to hold onto.

It is possible to recover from drug addiction. The tools needed to live a drug-free life are built and learned during treatment but once treatment is complete, addicts are not magically cured. Just as diabetics learn how to manage their diabetes, drug addicts can learn to manage their addiction. But, just like diabetics that chooses not to follow the diet that helps control their disease, drug addicts that fail to use those tools and skills to manage their disease will relapse. Recovery is possible but it is a commitment that requires attention and effort every day.

What Is America's #1 Addiction?

When addiction was just a moral failing or a self-centered, self-destructive choice, those who did not succumb to the allure of drugs, alcohol, or even cigarettes could feel confident that they had to develop moral fortitude or the strength of will to resist these unhealthy temptations. But the truth is, anyone can become an addict and the things we can become addicted to aren't limited to those three obvious addictive substances.

We humans can actually become addicted to just about anything, healthy or unhealthy, socially acceptable or unacceptable, moral or immoral. There is no real moral high ground upon which those who are not addicted to drugs, alcohol, or smoking can look down upon those who are because they may be addicts too; they just don't realize it yet because the things they are addicted to aren't vilified by society.

Addiction is a disease and anyone can get it. For example, the number one addiction in America today is addiction to prescription medication. While we have all heard the stories of teenagers stealing meds to use to get high; this is not the type of addiction referred to here.

This addiction is widespread and at the heart of it is our growing tendency to see every problem, every ailment, and every discomfort as something that can be solved by taking a pill. American medicine cabinets are full of drugs to help us manage our lives. There is Ambien to help us sleep, Xanax and Klonopin to ease our anxiety, Valium to keep us calm, and Vicodin and Oxycodone to take all our pain away.

From up on that moral high ground, most of the people who use these medications would never consider themselves addicts. Because these medications came from a doctor and are used to "treat" something, there is no moral judgment about taking them, even if they are taken when they aren't needed, even when they are taken longer than they should be.

But the statistics tell a different story. Across the country, deaths from drug overdose are the second leading cause of accidental death, right behind car accidents. And in some states, drug overdose has overtaken automobile accidents as the leading cause of accidental death.

But those deaths are not the result of the drugs we would expect like heroin, cocaine, or meth. These death rates are attributed to prescription drug overdoses because it is the use of the Ambien, the Xanax, the Klonopin, the Valium, the Vicodin, the Oxycodone and other prescription drugs to which so many people have become addicted that are killing more of us than anything other than car accidents.

Through the Eyes of Addiction

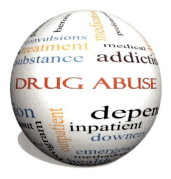

For those who have never experienced addiction, it can be impossible to understand the way it feels to be triggered, how strong and undeniable the cravings can be, and how little control an addict has when it comes to participating in the compulsive behaviors being demanded by the chemicals in their brain.

Changing the paradigm of addiction requires us to begin looking at addicts in a different way. Not as self-destructive, self-involved morally corrupt people who don't care about anything except for their next fix, but as people dealing with a chronic illness that, if untreated, is likely to kill them and who need the support, understanding, and accommodation given to others who are struggling with chronic disease.

This shift starts by opening our minds to understanding how the world looks through the eyes of addiction.

Walking the Dangerous Path - It's Not Your Fault

One person's addiction story resembles many cases I've seen. John tells the story of his addiction from a personal point of view:

I didn't start out with the intention to become an addict. I started drinking young and liked the way it felt to let the world fall away, but alcohol is hard to get and easy to detect, even if you use breath mints.

I tried weed which offered a different kind of world falling away feeling, it worked but I didn't want to chance getting caught – I needed to be able to let the world fall away when it got to be too much. Worrying about the smell, the papers, the bong was causing so much anxiety, I started thinking about giving it up.

That's when I took my first Perc...Percocet 10. I was at a party, wavering on whether or not to smoke up, worried about the smell but wanting that feeling. This guy offered one up, promising just what I wanted and that small, easy to hide pill delivered. I took another one the next weekend and it wasn't long before I was chipping in and helping to buy them myself. The beauty of this buzz was no smell, no papers, no bong, nothing but a tiny pill which made getting caught much less likely.

It didn't take long for that 10 to go to a 20 and even less time for the 20 to become a 30. Pills were perfect. Cheap, easy, and no telltale signs to give it away. But then I needed more than the people I was buying with which meant buying them on my own.

Pills operate on a kind of Costco model; the more you buy the cheaper each pill is. When you are buying with friends that works fine because everyone gets a cheaper price and there isn't a lot of extra hanging around. But now I was buying them on my own and I didn't want to pay $25 a pill. The answer was easy....I would buy 10 now instead of 1, have enough for the next couple weekends, and save money. I felt really smart.

But now, I had them on hand, and when Tuesday turned lopsided it was easy to rationalize popping that little pill and letting the world fall away for a little while. Especially because the voice in my brain assured me it was only going to be that once. This is how "on the weekends" became a "couple times a week".

The step from there to popping one in the morning like a vitamin was very small. At first, that one pill was enough for a bit of a buzz but then I needed it just to feel normal, just to function and go about my day. If I was stressed or anxious or depressed and needed that world falling away feeling, I had to take 2 or 3 or even 4 in a single day to get it.

This was the point that I realized I was spending all the money I had or made on percs. I decided I needed to cut back a little, curb my spending some, but that desire didn't even last a day. When my habit topped the $300 a week mark, I quickly began to run out of money. I couldn't pay for my car, I was on my last tank of gas, and didn't dare try to borrow any more money from any family members.

I was anxious and worried that my parents would realize my savings account was empty and depressed that I didn't have any money to buy the cute shoes at my favorite store when I popped the last 3 pills I had in my purse. I had a flash of anxiety that I didn't have any more pills that was rapidly washed away along with the rest of my worries as the drugs kicked in.

But then, that feeling wore off, reality started to come crashing down, and I almost unconsciously reached for the small box of safety I kept tucked away in my purse. Then I remembered that it was empty. I panicked and started calling around, trying to find someone I knew who had some to share. I begged the guy I bought them from to front me a few until Friday, but he just smiled and said cash only, no credit.

And as those first few hours became a day and that first day became two, the withdrawal set in and I began to entertain the idea of doing things I would never have even considered in order to get money to buy pills or to get the pills themselves.

I wish that was my version of what people call "rock bottom" but it was only a short stopover on my way down. Unfortunately, my journey to the bottom wasn't over, in some ways it was just beginning. As I called around, frantic, needing to not feel anything even for a few minutes just to get out from under the crushing effects of the withdrawal, I kept striking out until a friend of someone's friend said "I can't help with the percs right now but I have some smack that might help hold you over until you find some".

Part of my brain was shocked. Smack was heroin, heroin was for drug addicts, and I was not a drug addict. But the rest of my brain said pawn that necklace your grandma gave you so you can give him the $20 he needs so you can stop feeling like this, you will be able to figure things out better once you feel better.

As I felt the world falling away with that first hit of heroin I couldn't understand why I had spent so much time feeling horrible when I could have felt like this the whole time. Plus, heroin was so much cheaper, it seemed like an easy way to be okay while I got back on my feet and as long as I only used it for a couple days or maybe a week, I didn't have to worry about becoming an addict. At least, that is what the voice in my brain kept telling me.

The problem with heroin was that the same thing happened again. A little bump became a big bump which turned into a bag and before I knew it, my habit was back up to $200+ a week. Except now, it was heroin.

There wasn't any quick fix that could get me out of that jam. And those things I never thought I would do - the things that were unthinkable only a year ago started to seem like perfectly reasonable ways to get what I needed so that I could feel normal again. For me, the road ahead only had three destinations: jail, rehab, or death.

If you really want to keep kids off this path, you need to draw a very clear line between the pot and booze you don't want them to use and the dangerous drugs they need to avoid. Right now, alcohol, marijuana, cocaine, heroin, meth, bath salts, X, and whatever pills we can get our hands on are treated the same. They are all equally bad in the eyes of adults, law enforcement, and society in general. And this means that teenagers and young adults treat them as if they are the same. But they aren't the same.

Everyone needs to understand the difference between pot and alcohol, which can be addicting but which are not the same as opiates and heroin. Teenagers need to see what this path looks like and where it leads so they will know that popping percs on the weekend isn't the shortcut to the alcohol buzz they are looking for. They need to understand where this path leads and what it looks like and where to go for help if the find themselves on it. And we need places for them to go.

Right now, once you start down that path, you have nowhere to turn when you realize you are in trouble. You can't go to the cops because they will likely arrest you and you may end up with legal troubles. . You can't go to your doctor because they may lack the training, understanding and experience to help you. You can't go to your family because, well, you just can't. It's time to step off the moral high ground and take the steps that need to be taken to keep kids off this path and to help them early and effectively when that doesn't work.

Just Say No was the anti-drug mantra for almost two generations of children. It didn't work and now it's time to find something that will. Kids don't need mantras, they need honesty. They need information. They need to understand that smoking pot and shooting heroin is not the same thing and they need to understand why. And they need a safety net to catch them when they make bad decisions because they are teenagers and that's what teenagers do.

A True Story

Here's another example – a case I find often happens. Have you ever felt like this?

I don't know what to do. I am so scared and there is nowhere to turn for help, no one who understands what I am going through. No one to help. I just took the last three pills from my mom's night stand. I can't pretend any more than she isn't going to notice.

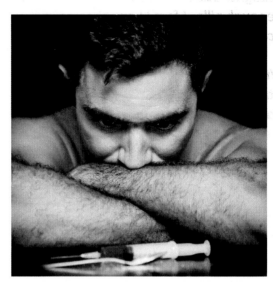

I tried not to, god did I try. I hate myself for doing it but it's like I am not in control of my own hands. I watch as my hand reaches for the bottle, removes the cap, sneaks out a few pills, and all the while there is a small voice in the back of my mind telling me it's wrong, yelling at me for stealing my mom's medication, cursing me for the horrible, worthless person I am. But even as that voice goes on and on, it never stops me from putting the pills in my mouth.

I love my mom so much. She is an amazing person and I know she would do anything for me but that doesn't stop me from stealing money from her purse. I hate myself more each time and I know she knows. She knows about the money and she knows about the pills, but she is ashamed and embarrassed and she doesn't know what to do either, so she doesn't say anything.

This is not who I am. This is not who I was supposed to be. This isn't the kind of thing that is supposed to happen to people like me. I am scared all the time. Scared of being caught. Scared of not being caught. Scared of taking too many pills. Scared I won't have enough pills. I fear I have become the kind of person I hate but I can't seem to stop it. I don't know what to do.

It's not like I am an **addict** *addict, you know? I mean, I am sure there are people who take a lot more than I do. And it's not like I am doing meth or shooting heroin or something bad like that. It's just Vicodin. It can't be that bad since it comes from a doctor. It's not like a real drug and I only take it because it smoothes out my edges; it makes my world work right. And I am not taking a lot, well, I take it every day but it's a low dosage.*

I am freaking out because I just took the last of the pills and I know my Mom is going to have to say something this time because she doesn't have any pills to take for her back. God, I am so stupid, why did I take the last three pills. She is going to have to say something because they aren't going to let her refill her prescription and now I don't know where I am going to get more. I don't know how I am going to get up tomorrow and make it through the day.

I am crying, hard, because I don't know how I got here. I can't stand to have my Mom look at me because of the sadness, loss, and regret in her eyes. She doesn't see me, she she's this monster that steals her money and steals her meds and she wonders what else I am doing to feed my habit. My habit. Oh god, I have a habit. I can't go a single day without chemical intervention. No wonder she hates me. Who wouldn't hate me? How did I get here?

I have to stop. I have to quit cold turkey. Enough is enough. I am not the kind of person that goes to rehab and I am not the kind of person who steals from my mother. I can't let everyone else in my life know what a mess I really am. They only see the outside, the external. They see the job, the friends, the dates, but they don't know that the only thing keeping me together is the same thing that is tearing me apart. I started taking the pills so I could feel nothing for a little while but now I have to take them to feel anything at all. I don't know how I got here. This isn't supposed to be my life. I have always been the good girl. I have a good job and yet, I steal money from my poor mother. What is wrong with me? I can't seem to stop crying. I have to do something but I don't even know where to start.

Opiate Dependence

What Can You Do With Prescription or Non Prescription Opiate Dependence?

This is the question many addicts find themselves asking at different points along that path. Overcoming opiate dependence is challenging and most addicts cannot do it on their own. While it is possible to have a spontaneous or instant remission or to quit cold turkey, most people need a program that combines different approaches to get clean and learn the skills they need to stay that way.

There is no one size fits all treatment plan that will work for every person who has an opiate addiction. Most programs combine biological assistance, psychological supports, and spirituality to find the best approach for the individual addict.

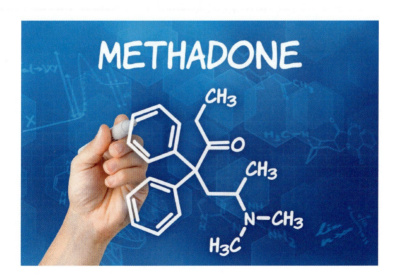

Biological Support

In terms of treating addiction, biological assistance generally comes in the form of a prescription medication. It includes identifying and simultaneously treating co-occurring disorders such as Attention Deficit Disorder, Bipolar Disorder, Anxiety Disorders, Depressive Disorders, Eating Disorders or Post Traumatic Disorder. Untreated psychiatric disorders are a critical reason for relapse as addicts tend to self-medicate unpleasant symptoms during periods of sobriety. Additional support to diagnose and treat Infectious diseases such as HIV, Hepatitis or Tuberculosis is integral to the overall treatment of the whole person.

This kind of comprehensive disease management must be provided by a doctor and medications must be administered under their supervision. Medication may be provided as part of an inpatient program or as a doctor supervised outpatient program.

The goal of using medication as part of an overall treatment plan for addiction is to slow down or cool off the dopamine pathways that are part of the brain's reward system. Medication has traditionally accomplished this in two different ways.

It either "feeds the beast in a regulated and controlled manner" by supplementing the chemical reaction usually experienced when using drugs in an effort to eliminate the cravings that lead to the compulsion to use. Or it blocks the receptors in the brain that are activated during drug use so that the addict doesn't experience anything if they do use. With this approach, over time, the brain should stop craving the drug because it isn't getting the payoff that it used to get.

There is a new approach that combines the two traditional methods to help with both withdrawal and cravings. This kind of medication blocks most of the receptors so using drugs doesn't produce the expected effect but it doesn't block all of them. By allowing a small amount to be activated, this kind of medication helps calm the cravings as well.

There are three medications that are used to aid in treating opiate addiction. Each of these medications produces one of the results outlined above.

Methadone

What is it?
Methadone which also goes under the names Amidone, Dolophine, Heptadon, Methadose, Physeptone, and Symoron, among others, is a synthetically created opioid used to treat opioid dependence. It is also used to treat severe chronic pain.

How does it help?
Methadone is the prescription medication used to "feed the beast" of opiate addiction. It acts on the same receptors in the brain as other opiate drugs and provides a similar, albeit longer, effect. When taken orally, it can help eliminate or reduce cravings for other opiates and decrease the symptoms of withdrawal addict's experience.

If given at a high enough dose, methadone also blocks the pleasurable effects provided by other opiates. For some addicts, methadone makes it possible to decrease or cease their use of other opiate substances.

How to get it?

Traditionally, methadone is dispensed as part of an outpatient program through a methadone clinic under the supervision of a physician. These clinics are highly regulated and initially patients are required to come to the clinic every day to get their medication and must be observed taking it on the premises.

While this requirement can become less restrictive over time, it is important in the initial stages to tightly control access and monitor compliance to ensure addicts don't swap one addiction for another. Addicts who obtain methadone from a clinic may also be required to pass drug screens in order to continue receiving the medication.

Buprenorphine

What is it?

Buprenorphine, which is also called Suboxone or Zubsolvis a semi-synthetic partial opioid agonist used to treat addiction to opiates.

How does it help?

Buprenorphine helps addicts learn to manage their addiction by doing two things. First, it blocks most of the receptors in the brain that respond to the use of opiates. This means that if the addict uses, they will not get the expected effect.

Over time, this helps undo some of the hardwiring in the brain caused by the addiction and eliminates the craving for the drug. Second, unlike Naltrexone which blocks all these receptors, this medication allows some of the receptors to be activated which provides enough opiate-like effect to calm the cravings, similar to what methadone does but on a smaller scale.

These two effects together help eliminate or reduce the cravings while working to reverse the addiction hardwiring in the brain in an effort to make disease management easier over the long term.

How to get it?
A physician can prescribe buprenorphine for you but only physicians who have taken special training are certified to prescribe it. You will need to find a physician who is able to prescribe it. It comes in a pill and can generally be taken at home.

Naltrexone

What is it?
Naltrexone which is also called Revia, Depade, and Vivitrol is an opioid receptor antagonist that blocks the effects of opiates in the brain. It is used to treat both alcohol and opioid dependence.

How does it help?
Naltrexone blocks the receptors in the brain that are activated when a person uses an opiate like heroin. By blocking these receptors, the medication keeps the addict from experiencing the euphoric effects of the opiate. It does not treat, effect or eliminate the craving for the drug, only the effect the addict experiences. The goal of using this drug is to eliminate the cravings over time by convincing the brain there is no pleasurable payoff of taking them.

How to get it?
Naltrexone can be provided in a pill or in an intramuscular injection. It has to be prescribed by a physician and may be provided as part of an inpatient or outpatient substance abuse program or by your primary care physician.

Psychological Support

In addition to medication, treating drug addiction generally requires

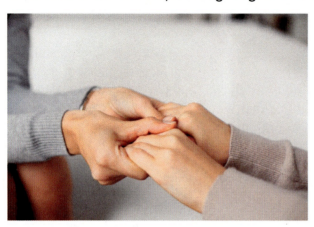

psychological support as well. This kind of support can include traditional cognitive behavioral therapy, mindfulness training, and the use of specific programs developed to meet the psychological needs of drug addicts in recovery.

This kind of support can be provided on an inpatient or outpatient basis using a variety of programs.

Intensive Outpatient Program (IOP)

This type of program is used to treat all forms of chemical dependency but it does not deal with detoxification. The addicts who participate in this kind of psychological support program don't require the same level of comprehensive care needed by those in more intensive programs. Most IOP programs utilize a combination of group and individual therapeutic techniques.

Participants will spend 10-12 hours per week receiving services. For many addicts, this kind of program is ideal because the lack of a residential component and the limited time commitment required make it possible to engage in normal activities like holding down a job or caring for loved ones while still participating in the program. Sessions and services may be scheduled in the early mornings, evenings, and on weekends to accommodate participants.

In addition to the services provided as part of the program itself, most IOPs also encourage or require participation in a 12 step program. IOPs may also be used as a way to transition addicts from a rehabilitation facility or a PHP back to a completely independent living situation.

Partial Hospitalization Program (PHP)

Partial hospitalization or PHP allows participants to continue living at home but provides a comprehensive program at a hospital that may require participant attendance 7 days a week. This type of program is aimed at reducing the number of people who require inpatient care and reducing the overall cost of long-term care.

 The focus of PHP is to treat the whole person and is designed to meet the needs of those who need more intensive care than provided in an IOP or an Office-Based program but who do not need to or cannot be away from their home and family 24 hours a day. PHP includes group and individual therapy, skill building, psycho-education sessions, and psychopharmacological assessment, administration, and monitoring.

Comprehensive Inpatient or Residential Program (Rehab)
This type of program is what most people traditionally think of as rehab. It provides the same types of care as a PHP but participates live at the treatment facility or hospital for the length of the program. Many residential programs begin with detoxification and generally last 28, 30, or 90 days.

Cognitive Behavioural Therapy (CBT)

Regardless of what kind of program an addict participates in, they are likely to take part in cognitive behavioral therapy in both individual and group settings. CBT is a type of talk therapy that helps participants identify how their thoughts influence their behavior, specifically addressing unhealthy, negative, and irrational thoughts.

Research has shown that unhealthy patterns of thinking are always present with addiction, regardless of what kind of addiction a person has. These thought patterns play a role in the development of the addiction, and breaking that negative thought pattern cycle is how addicts use new beneficial behaviors to replace the unhealthy behaviors that initiated and enabled their addiction.

Individual Cognitive Therapy
Individual cognitive therapy involves 1 on 1 meetings between a therapist and an addict. During these sessions, the therapist helps the addict identify the negative thought patterns and difficult emotions that are at the route of their addiction. For most addicts, the use of drugs begins as a means for escaping these negative thoughts and feelings. Understanding the unhealthy thought patterns that opened the door to addiction helps the therapist and addict replace them with positive thoughts.

Learning to focus on positive thinking and learning to deal with underlying emotions can help build self-esteem and effect positive change on thought patterns. These skills, in turn, make the addict more resilient and increase the confidence they have in themselves and their ability to handle everyday situations without becoming overwhelmed and use positive, healthy coping skills when difficulties arise rather than resorting to their previous destructive behavior patterns.

Individual CBT can also be beneficial for recovering addicts because it supports the gradual process necessary for overcoming addiction. The 1 on 1 nature of this relationship allows for the process to move at the speed most appropriate for the addict and makes it possible to tailor each session to the individual's specific needs.

This kind of CBT is especially beneficial for addicts who have a dual diagnosis. These people must learn to overcome addiction while managing another mental health condition like depression or anxiety.

Group Cognitive Behavioural Therapy
Group CBT uses the same foundational principles and practices of individual CBT but in a group setting. Groups are generally made up of addicts with similar addictions or who are in similar stage in their recovery.

There is a symbiotic relationship between individual CBT and group CBT sessions. The easiest way to understand it is that individual CBT helps identify and build the skills needed to overcome negative thought patterns, build resilience and self-esteem, and manage the disease. Group CBT provides an arena in which to practice, test, and refine those new skills.

Additionally, group CBT helps addicts understand and learn to deal with peer pressure. This kind of influence often plays a role in the initial stages of drug use and in the development and perpetuation of the addiction. Overcoming and learning to manage the addiction requires that addicts build the skills, confidence, and resilience to withstand the powerful force that peer pressure can apply.

Because the group session involves peer to peer and interpersonal interactions, it provides the perfect opportunity to practice these new skills and build up confidence in their ability to resist participating when faced with a real life situation.

Another benefit of group CBT is that is builds a sympathetic support network of other addicts who have similar experiences, have gone through the same program, and who are working towards the same goal. This support network can be crucial to helping individuals navigate challenging times that may have ended in a relapse without the positive thoughts and encouragement the group setting can provide.

This kind of CBT is generally included in every kind of addiction recovery program and is often the final stage of support once addicts are clean and sober, and working to maintain their sobriety.

Mindfulness Based Approaches

Mindfulness is a form of meditation that encourages present awareness, acceptance of thoughts and feelings without judgment, acknowledgement of physical sensations and mental noise, and recognition that all these experiences are fleeting and temporary in nature.

 It is a specific way of paying attention to what is going on around you and inside you that focuses on acknowledgement and acceptance rather than modification and suppression. The focus on acceptance of thoughts and feelings rather than suppression is one of the reasons mindfulness based training and supportive therapies are being effectively used to help treat those with substance abuse problems.

Based on research supporting the theory that a mindfulness based approach can be effective in preventing drug abuse relapse, mindfulness programs and therapeutic methods have been developed to address the specific needs of this population.

Other approaches designed to help address mental health conditions like Mindfulness-Based Cognitive Therapy (MBCT), Dialectical Behavior Therapy (DBT), and Acceptance and Commitment Therapy (ACT) have been modified for use in substance abuse recovery programs. These modified approaches include Mindfulness-Based Relapse Prevention (MBRP) and Mindfulness-Based Therapeutic Community (MBTC) treatment.

The way mindfulness training and meditation benefits individuals with addiction is by helping them identify and understand what drives their cravings and new ways of managing the discomfort unappeased cravings can create. Where traditionally, the addict would have turned to drugs in order to cope with difficult emotions, they can use these new skills to acknowledge and accept unpleasant thoughts and feelings rather than avoiding them and interrupt their habitual response patterns using present awareness.

New research indicates that post-recovery support programs that incorporate mindfulness based training can be more effective than other, more traditional, treatment approaches at preventing drug abuse relapse over the long term.

SMART

SMART Recovery® (Self-Management And Recovery Training) is an addiction recovery support group that helps participants learn the tools they need to maintain their recovery over the long term. SMART Recovery® is a 4 point program that uses the latest research from the scientific community to support recovery from all different kinds of addictions. Those in the program attend face-to-face meetings, online meetings, and communicate with each other via message boards and chat rooms.

SMART Recovery® differs from some of the more familiar 12 step addiction support programs in some important ways. Where many of the 12 step programs are built around a center of spirituality, the SMART Recovery® program is built around a scientific center. Understanding, discussing, and incorporating the latest scientific research about addiction is a core differentiator of the program. SMART Recovery® also focus on building a sense of self-reliance and avoids using labels that can make participants feel limited and powerless.

The 4-Point Program offers specific tools and techniques for each of the program points:

Step 1: Building and Maintaining Motivation
Step 1 of SMART Recovery® program is all about empowering those who are dealing with addiction to decide if they are ready to make the changes needed to learn to manage their addiction.

Once the decision is made, the program supports that decision by helping the individual build the motivation necessary to make the change and to maintain their motivation throughout the process. One of the techniques used in step 1 is called motivational interviewing.

It involves two participants, a care provider and a client. It is a collaborative effort where the care provider and the client work together to discuss the motivation to change, discuss any reasons the client has for not deciding to change, and exchanging perspectives based on their own individual strengths and experiences.
SMART Recovery® is based around the idea that the first step an addict has to take on the road to recovery and addiction management is to make the conscious choice to do so. This first step empowers clients to embrace this position of power over their own lives.

The step uses techniques like motivational interviewing to help them navigate through the avoidance, denial, rationalization, and other tactics everyone uses when faced with a difficult challenge so that they can find their own motivation and build it up so that it can maintain them through the difficult steps ahead.   Here is an example of what this looks like.

Mike grew up in Minnesota and struggled with anxiety since he was a teenager. He turned to drug use as a way to cope with his anxiety. The combination of his drug use and his anxiety made him difficult to be around. He was very distant, engaging only in surface-level interactions, and came across as distrustful and paranoid around other people.

Mike would drop in on meetings erratically, but wasn't willing to commit to the program, to see any specialists, or to accept any support. He was afraid of being medicated. He was convinced that accepting help meant relinquishing his rights and he didn't trust any organized system, government or not.

Joe, one of the care providers, had tried on numerous occasions to develop a connection with Mike to no avail. Then, one day, Joe saw Mike digging around in a pile of trash behind a shopping center. He stopped and slowly approached Mike, hoping he may be more receptive away from the program.

Mike offered Joe a genuine smile when he saw him, the first one Joe had ever seen, and motioned him over to see something sitting with a dirty backpack.

Joe knew immediately what he was looking at, even though to most people it would have looked like a beat-up old military helmet. Joe smiled back and started asking Mike questions about the helmet. They quickly realized that they had a shared love for World War II memorabilia which created the kind of connect Joe had been trying to build all along.

Through this shared interest, Joe was able to help Mike open up. Over time, through their discussions about WWII memorabilia, Mike was able to start sharing his thoughts and feelings about other parts of his life. As Joe got to know Mike better, he was able to expand their conversations and through the use of motivational interviewing use their connection and shared interests to help Mike take the first steps toward recovery.

Step 2: Coping With Urges
It is normal for addicts, even those in recovery, to experience cravings and compulsive urges. Early in the recovery process these cravings and urges can be very intense and difficult to manage. They may even seem impossible to ignore.

Arming clients with more than a dozen strategies for coping with cravings and urges until they pass is step 2 of the SMART Recovery® program. By creating a plan for how they will cope with these inevitable discomforts, clients are prepared to live with the uncomfortable feelings until they pass and become more resilient and less likely to relapse.

One of the coping strategies from the SMART Recovery® program that can be beneficial in helping clients cope with cravings and urges is called DEADS. It stands for:

- Delay – Because cravings and urges are short-lived discomforts, they will disappear if they aren't sustained by our attention. Delaying gratification of the urge until it passes helps build muscle memory that will make it easier to delay gratification the next time and the time after that.
- Escape – Vacate the area and get away from whatever is triggering the craving and urge to participate in addictive behavior. Simply changing location or scenery can often be enough to shift the focus away from the urge to use.

- Accept – Accepting that overcoming addiction can be uncomfortable and then accepting the discomfort of the craving or urge in the moment is another way to cope. Many addicts use drugs to alleviate discomfort and learning to live with unpleasant experiences and sensations is a critical skill on the road to long term recovery.
- Dispute – Have an argument with yourself as a way of coping with irrational urges. Preparing logical arguments ahead of time provides the ammunition necessary to counteract the irrational arguments being presented by the addiction. This internal dispute can provide a distraction that will help the craving or urge dissipate more quickly.
- Substitute – Another way of coping is to immediately swap in some other thought or activity for the craving whenever an urge rears its unpleasant head. You might picture your happy place or go for a walk or listen to a favorite song. The key is to replace the unpleasant cravings and urge with something positive and empowering.

Step 3: Managing Thoughts, Feelings and Behaviors
Experts have long understood that negative thought patterns and unpleasant feelings are at the heart of addictive behavior. For most people struggling with addiction, the choice to use drugs in the first place was a maladaptive coping strategy for dealing with difficult emotions.

The third step invites clients to learn new ways to manage their thoughts, feelings, and behaviors using rational thinking. The techniques used in this step help clients challenge the negative thoughts and feelings they are experiencing and then use healthier, more positive thoughts and feelings that are based on rational thought to replace them.

One of the techniques used in this step is called Rational Emotive Behavior Therapy (REBT). It is a type of CBT that teaches the client to do this kind of thought swap.

By learning to identify, confront, and consciously change the self-harming, defeatist thought patterns and belief systems into healthier, more productive ones, clients learn how to increase their own emotional well-being, practice setting and achieving goals in the short term, and gain confidence in their ability to achieve longer term goals.

The ABCs of REBT is one of the tools used to achieve this kind of thought and behavior modification. The emphasis here, as well as in other areas of the program, is on using self-discipline and self-motivation as the client accepts personal responsibility for being the driving force behind ending their addictive behavior.   Here are the ABCs of REBT:

Activating Event – The activating event is the "thing" that happened that brought forth the negative thoughts or feelings that must be managed. Identifying the activating event is an important part of the process. Clients learn to ask themselves questions like:
- What happened that brought these feelings or beliefs to the surface?
- Was it something I did?
- Was it something done by something else?
- Was it a person, place, thing, sound, or smell?
- Was it a thought or idea in my own head?

An example of an activating event would be thinking about your boyfriend who also uses drugs.

Beliefs - The next step is to challenge and analyze the beliefs the client has about the activating event. The analysis helps them determine whether or not the things they believe are actually true. Clients learn to ask themselves questions like:

- What do I believe about this event?
- What do I think is true about this event?
- What am I telling myself?
- Are these beliefs helpful?
- Are these beliefs self-defeating?

An example of this kind of belief is that if you aren't doing drugs too, he won't love you anymore and if you don't want to lose him, you must do drugs too.

Consequence – The next step is to examine how you feel about those beliefs and to identify how you would normally react when you experience those feelings. Clients learn to ask themselves questions like:

- How does this make me feel?
- Am I feeling anger?
- Anxiety?
- Frustration?
- Hopelessness?
- How would I react normally?
- Do these feelings cause negative behaviors?

An example of this kind of consequence would be: "Thinking about losing my boyfriend makes me feel anxious, fearful, unloved, and alone. When I experience these kinds of negative emotions taking drugs makes me feel better."

Disputing Irrational Beliefs– The final step is to use the information gathered to dispute the validity of the beliefs about the event that are untrue, irrational, or dysfunctional. Clients learn to ask themselves questions like:

- Is the belief I have about that activating event helpful?

- Is the belief I have about that activating event self-defeating?
- Is this belief realistic?
- Is this belief logical?
- Is this belief rational?
- Does the event warrant the severity of my beliefs; is it bad enough to make me believe such negative things?

An example of how clients can dispute these irrational beliefs using the example above can look like this.

- Will my boyfriend really stop loving me if I stop taking drugs?
- Do I actually want to be in a relationship with someone who is using if I am working hard not to use?
- Do I think it is realistic to believe I can stay clean if I remain in a relationship with someone who is using?

New Effect or Rational Belief - Once the client has disputed their beliefs about the event and sorted rational, reasonable beliefs from irrational, unhealthy beliefs, they can identify new rational beliefs to replace the irrational beliefs about that event. Clients learn to ask themselves questions like:

- What new rational belief can I use to replace each irrational belief?
- How does this change how I feel about the event?
- How will this change the consequences?

An example of a new, rational belief could be if my boyfriend loves me, he should want what is best for me and if I believe that being clean is what is best for me, he will support my decision to be clean and my efforts to live without drugs.

If he doesn't support my decision, it is because he doesn't love me or he isn't strong enough to support what is best for me, either of which mean he isn't a good partner for me. I will be hurt and sad, but I can handle those emotions because I know that I am choosing what is right for me and if he is not right for me, it is not because I am unlovable or worthless and it doesn't mean I will be alone forever.

Laid out this way it may seem like working through the ABCs is a straight forward, relatively easy process. But changing thought patterns that have deep roots and that have been in place for a long time is not as easy as asking a few questions and deciding to think differently. This is a process that takes time, practice, commitment, and perseverance.

Dysfunctional beliefs, irrational thoughts, and self-destructive behaviors are not going to be changed overnight. Understanding that and expecting these kinds of changes to take time helps keep people from becoming frustrating and giving up.

While the ABCs tool is taught as a way to help manage urges and cravings it can actually be used in any situation where negative thoughts pop up, unhealthy feelings arise, or destructive behaviors feel imminent. It is a powerful tool for developing self-acceptance that many people learn to use across many areas of their life. It encourages the establishment of the belief that you can only change your own thinking and your own behavior and you are the only one that can change those things.

Step 4: Living A Balanced Life

The fourth step in the SMART Recovery® program seeks to help clients understand what it means to them to live a balanced life and learn to make choices that create that balance.

From the perspective of the program, balance is about making peace with the difference between instant and delayed gratification and knowing when each applies. Achieving this kind of balance is crucial to relapse prevention.

Addiction is all about instant gratification which is why it is important to learn how to delay gratification as part of the recovery program. But swinging too far the other way is also unhealthy because if everything we do is about meeting long term needs, we miss out on the things we want to do that bring happiness and fulfillment now. Finding the balance between those two extremes is the essence of life balance.

Here is what balanced living can look like for a person who is managing their addiction.

At one point, when I was doing an inpatient program for my heroin addiction, I listened to a speaker who was talking about the importance of living a life that was balanced. The words sounded great, but in truth, they fell on deaf ears. I was still too close to a like centered on drug abuse to see how this balanced life idea could ever apply to me. I couldn't really grasp how this idea of life balance was going to help me stay clean and sober once I went home.

That was 8 years ago and now, with that many years clean and sober, I not only get why balanced living matters to those struggling with addiction, I can tell you that it is one of the foundational elements of my clean and sober life. You may be feeling like I did, all those years ago and wondering, yeah, but how does that help me where I am now. Here is what I learned as I made my way down my clean and sober path.

One of the interesting things that happen when you stay clean and sober is that your life starts to fill up. When you are using, everything is centered on that single aspect of your life. It fills up all the room in your life and there isn't any room for anything else. But when you are clean, your life opens up and there is space that can be filled by other things like friends and relationships and hobbies. In many ways, my using life was simple and my clean and sober life became more and more complex over time.

Good things happen and you grow and you learn new things and it can seem like there are so many things to do and see and learn and buy…..and it can become overwhelming. As your recovery life fills up, the need to have some kind of balance becomes critical to maintaining your recovery and all of the good things that are happening.

The fourth step in the SMART Recovery® program encourages clients to take all the skills they have learned and the tools they have used and apply them to defining short and long term goals that will help them find some kind of balance across the different areas of their life. Some of the considerations that are part of this process include:

- **Regaining Health** – Many of those who are recovering from addiction have suffered from poor health because of their drug use, poor health habits, and limited access to or willingness to use medical care. This means that one of the most important areas that many people need to set short- and long-term goals around is regaining their health. This can mean learning to eat a well-balanced diet, improving their sleep hygiene, and getting regular exercise.
- **Relaxation** – Mindfulness meditation is very beneficial for those in recovery from drug addiction and it, and other relaxation techniques, can be instrumental in helping people manage urges, overcome cravings, and reduce anxiety.

- **Goal Setting** –Setting goals for the short- and long-term that enable a person to achieve the things they want to do without neglecting the things they need to do is critical to finding the balanced lifestyle that is best for them. People are encouraged to focus on setting goals that are specific, realistic, measurable, and time-bound.
- **Social and Recreational Activities** –Becoming involved in things that are interesting and connecting with new people who will be part of the new life they are building are important ways to find joy and pleasure in the short and long term. Finding ways to support their belief that living a clean and sober life can be fulfilling, rewarding, and fun helps reaffirm that they do not have to participate in addictive behaviors.
- **Relapse Prevention**-Supporting their own recovery by defining strategies for preventing relapse can help those in recovery to keep from slipping backward and re-engaging in unhealthy behaviors.

This step encourages clients to embrace that the following components help to create and support a happy, healthy, balanced life.

- **Self-Acceptance:** Unconditional acceptance of who you are and letting go of the idea that you must prove yourself to others
- **Taking Risks:** Being open to taking emotional risks, being open to adventure, reaching for goals, but not being reckless, irrational, or self-destructive
- **Being Realistic:** Having a realistic expectation about what recovery is like including the fact that there will be rough patches, painful experiences, failures, and unachievable

desires and that the way forward involves recognizing these situations and not letting them push you off the path

- **High Tolerance for Frustration:** Understanding that there will always be things we can change and there will always be things we can't, and the only ones we should be focused on are the ones we can impact
- **Self-Responsibility:** Knowing that we are responsible for our own actions and that the responsibility for our thoughts, feelings, emotions, and actions lies only with us and no one else bears the blame for the bad things in our lives
- **Self-Interest:** Knowing that being available and helping others is important but that taking care of ourselves and tending to our own needs is more important
- **Social Interest:** Accepting that people are social creatures and that we need to be part of a social group with social interaction and understanding that we must seek out the groups and people who have the same values as we do
- **Self-Direction:** Accepting that we are solely responsible for our own lives and not dependent on the support of others
- **Tolerance**: Accepting that we are all human and that everyone makes mistakes and then being able to forgive when appropriate
- **Flexibility**: Being able to think openly, accept other ideas, and avoid holding others to strict ideals
- **Acceptance of Uncertainty**: Understanding that there will always be unknowns and that, despite this, you can live an ordered life that allows you to adjust to changing circumstances)

Spiritual Support

One of the most well-known recovery support programs for those who are addicted to drugs is Narcotics Anonymous. NA is a spiritual

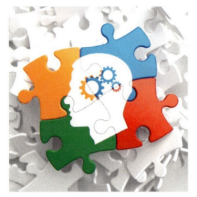

program that helps recovering addicts to develop their individual relationship with their higher power. The definition of what or who that higher power might be is open to the individual interpretation of each person in the program. For this reason, NA meetings are attended by people of all different faiths and belief systems.

Narcotics Anonymous is a 12 step program and each of the steps is based on a spiritual principle or ideal. For example, the first three steps encompass the spiritual principles of being honest, being open-minded, and being willing. By following these principles, NA members can create a path away from addiction and towards their new clean and sober life.

The spiritual nature of NA is also expressed in the way the meetings are run, where judgment is left outside the meeting and given over to the higher power. Anonymity is a core component of the program and part of its spiritual foundation. It is a constant reminder to members to "place principles before personalities" and that no member is ever superior to another member. Each meeting ends with a closing prayer like the serenity prayer most commonly associated with 12 step programs.

"God, Grant us the serenity to accept the things we cannot change, the courage to change the things we can, and the wisdom to know the difference."

The primary message of NA is that there is hope, that addiction can be managed, that recovery is possible. The 12 steps are the foundation for the promise that NA makes to its membership which is that "an addict, any addict, can stop using drugs, lose the desire to use, and learn a new way of life."

The NA program is comprised of three primary aspects: meetings, sponsors, and service.

Meetings are held in two formats, open and closed. Anyone can attend an open meeting at any time. Closed meeting attendance is limited to addicts and people who think they may be addicts. During each meeting, sometime is devoted to reading from NA literature out loud that touch on issues and concerns related to clean living.

Many meetings also feature a time for "open sharing" when attendees can get up and share stories and personal experiences related to their addiction, recovery, and overall process. This part of the meeting is not interactive and only one person speaks at a time.

Meetings can also be run in a round-robin format where people take turns speaking and sharing, similar to the format of a group therapy session. Meetings may also include time for a speaker, specific reading and discussion related to one of the 12 steps, and time for recognizing important milestones like clean time anniversaries.

Service is considered to be a critical part of an individual's recovery. In the NA context, services means "doing the right thing for the right reason." The type of service work varies from group to group. Examples of service include acting as the chair for a meeting, setting up before or cleaning up after a meeting, acting as the treasurer or secretary for the group, and acting as the Group Service Representative (GSR) that represents the group in the larger NA organization.

Sponsorship is an essential component of the NA program which pairs an experienced NA member with a new NA member in order to provide a designated source of guidance, mentoring, and support. Sponsors share their experiences, strategies, wisdom, and strength as they guide the other member through the 12 step program.

You Can Do It

Save Your Health, Save Your Life

Addiction is a disease of the brain. If you are addicted to using drugs it isn't because you are lazy, worthless, or a bad person. It is because you have an illness, an illness that can be treated.

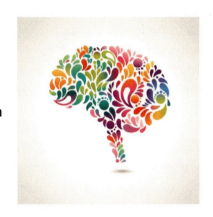

This means that you can get better, you can live without drugs, and you can experience all the wonderful things life has to offer. You can do it, and you are the only one that can do it.

The increased research understanding of what is happening in an addicted brain highlights the need to not only eliminate the use of drugs but also to do the work necessary to re-wire the pathways in your brain that have been hijacked by your addiction. This means choosing to pursue a clean and sober life is only the start of your journey down the path to living clean and being in control of your addiction.

Along the way you will need to develop new skills, open your mind to new ideas, and be willing to accept and move past failures and disappointments, and commit to continuing to work at being clean until you are. It won't be easy and it is important to understand that so that you expect bumps in the road and unplanned detours through the woods as part of your journey, and you don't allow them to derail your progress or give you a reason to give up.

One of the most challenging parts of your journey will be learning to identify the triggers that cause cravings and urges for the drugs you are trying to leave behind you. Knowing what makes you want to use makes it possible for you to challenge the negative thought patterns and irrational beliefs that support and feed the addiction.

Challenging the thoughts, feelings, and behaviors that feed the addiction make it possible to change how you respond to them. Learning to do these things takes the power for controlling your behavior away from the addiction and puts it back in your hands.

There are three primary sources of support along the path from addiction to a clean life.

- Biological Support which comes in the form of cutting edge evidence-based medications that can help to curb cravings and assist in rewiring the brain. It includes addressing treatment of co-occurring psychiatric disorders that might have been the reason to self-medicate with street drugs or have developed since the use of street drugs.
- Psychological Support which can be provided in different settings and can include individual or group therapy, mindfulness based training, and recovery support programs like the SMART Recovery® program.
- Spiritual Support which is most often provided by a 12 step program like Narcotics Anonymous.

It is possible to recover from drug addiction and live a clean, happy, hopeful life. The most effective way to stop using is to face your addiction and seek out the kinds of support you need to learn to control your addiction. A program that combines aspects from each of the three sources of support outlined here offers the best chance for a long-term recovery. You can learn how to use the tools, strategies, and skills you need to live a drug-free life. But you must always remember that there is no magic cure for addiction. Recovery is possible but it requires commitment, attention, and effort every day.

No matter what got you to where you are today, you have the power to save your life, to regain your health, and to reclaim your life from the addiction that is ruining it. The choice is yours, and you are the only one that can make it.

I wish you all success in your endeavors to beat your addiction and live the life you are meant to live!

Works Cited

"Addiction Is a Chronic Disease." NIDA. N.p., n.d. Web. 09 May 2014.

Brower, Vicki. "Summary." National Center for Biotechnology Information. U.S. National Library of Medicine, 25 Sept. 0005. Web. 07 May 2014.

"David Sheff: Drug Addiction Is a Disease - but a Curable One."

Fiore, Kristina. "Addictions, Bad Habits Can 'Highjack' Brain." ABC News. ABC News Network, 31 Jan. 2010. Web. 07 May 2014.

"Methadone Withdrawal Symptoms." Michaels House. N.p., n.d. Web. 07 May 2014.

Narcotics Anonymous. "What is the Narcotics Anonymous Program?". http://www.na.org. Narcotics Anonymous World Services, Inc. Web. 07 May 2014.

National Post Full Comment David Sheff Drug Addiction Is a Disease but a Curableone Comments. N.p., n.d. Web. 07 May 2014.

"Naltrexone for the Treatment of Alcohol Dependence among African Americans: Results from the COMBINE Study." Naltrexone for the Treatment of Alcohol Dependence among African Americans: Results from the COMBINE Study. N.p., n.d. Web. 07 May 2014.

"Recognizing Alcohol & Drug Addiction : The Effects of Withdrawal From Addiction." YouTube. YouTube, 20 Dec. 2007. Web. 07 May 2014.

"SMART Recovery." Drugs Forum RSS. N.p., n.d. Web. 07 May 2014.

Treatment, Center For Substance Abuse. National Center for Biotechnology Information. U.S. National Library of Medicine, 18 Apr. 0000. Web. 07 May 2014.

"Top 5 Addictions in the U.S." ADDICT NATION. N.p., n.d. Web. 07 May 2014.

"Why Therapy Is Essential in Treating Addiction." WebMD. WebMD, n.d. Web. 07 May 2014.

Made in the USA
Las Vegas, NV
05 November 2020